MW01248616

TOOTH LOVE

By Deveda Jackson
Illustrated by Brianna Osaseri

Print ISBN: 979-8-9863831-0-1

Ordering Information:
For details, contact deveda.jackson@gmail.com.

Printed by IngramSpark.

First printing edition 2022.

Design and editing credit: CLW Tucker | A Belief and Branding Agency, LLC www.clwtucker.com, info@clwtucker.com, (800) 840-9450

Illustrated by Brianna Osaseri.

This book is dedicated to:

To my husband, my father, and my two children.
Thank you for inspiring me to share my love of dentistry with the world!

Thank You

I love my teeth.
I need them to speak.
I love my teeth.
They shape my face-so neat!

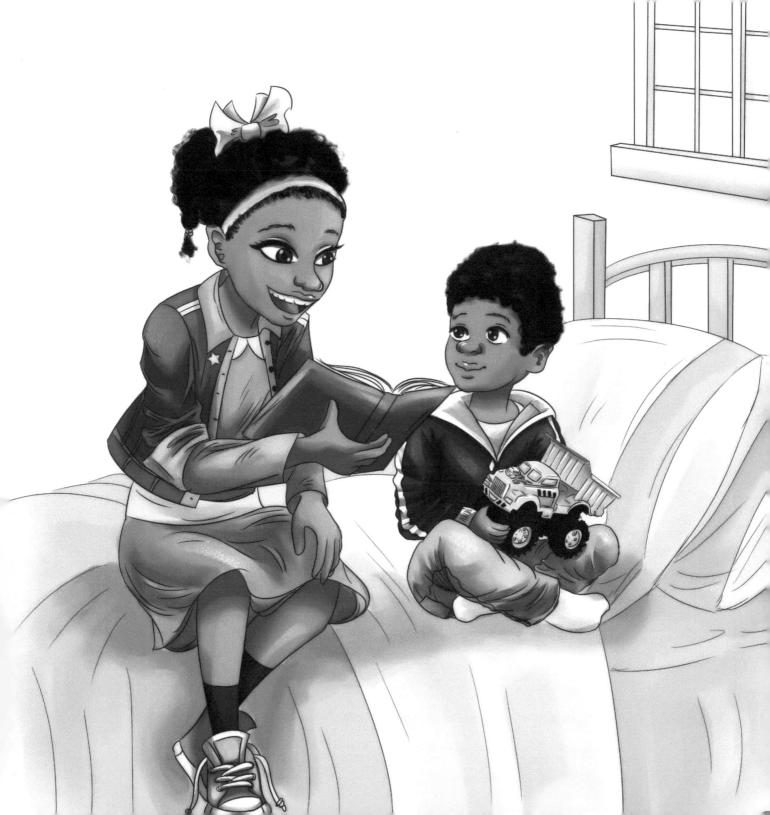

I love my teeth.
I brush them twice a day.
I love my teeth.
A little toothpaste goes a long way!

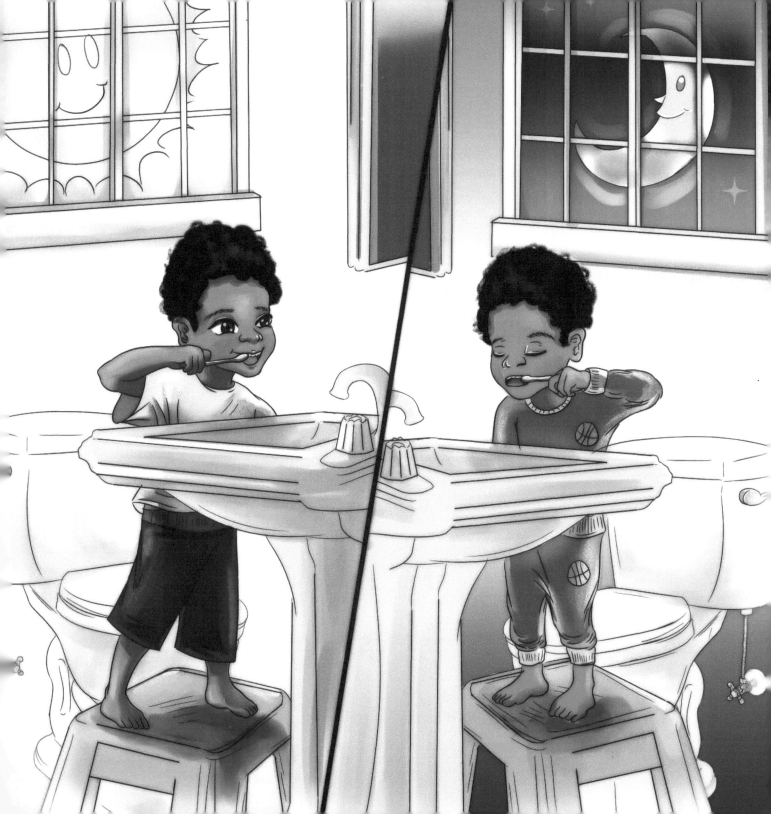

I love my teeth.
A soft toothbrush works the best.
I love my teeth.
Brushing makes my mouth fresh.

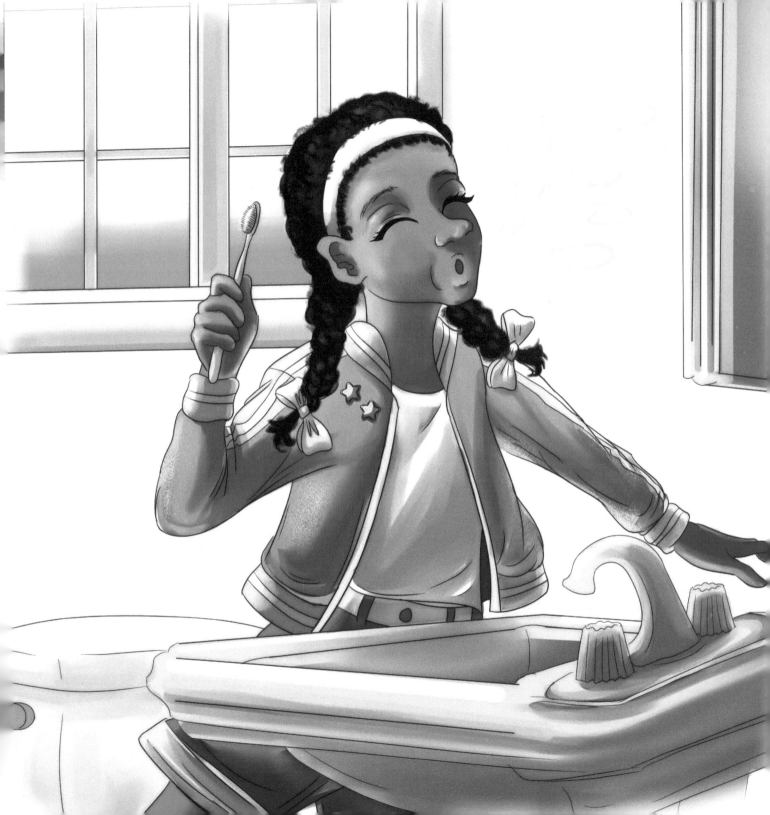

I love my teeth.
Brushing them in circles is what I do.
I love my teeth.
I brush not one minute but two!

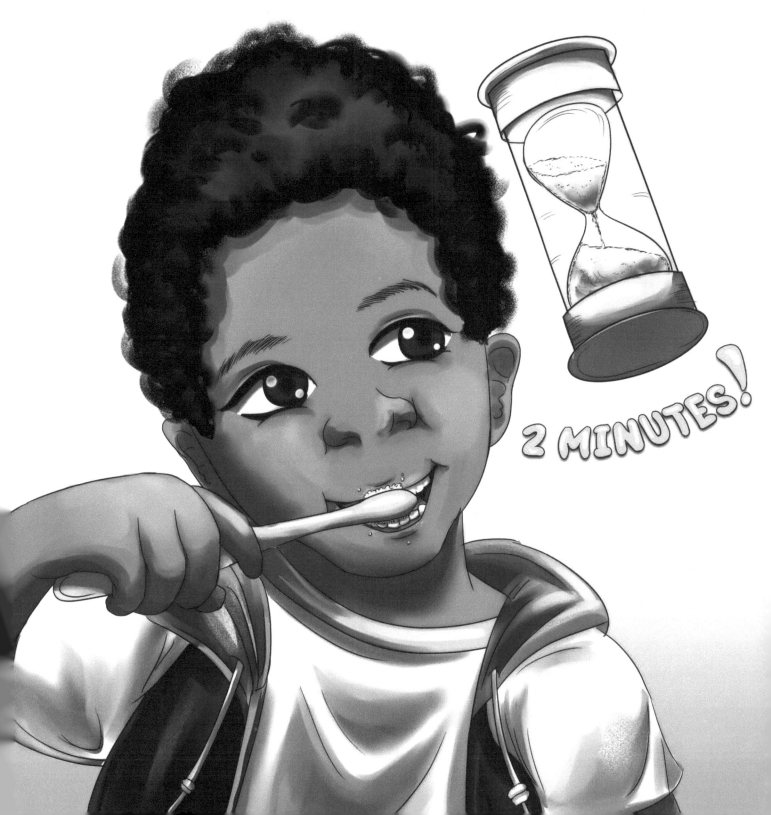

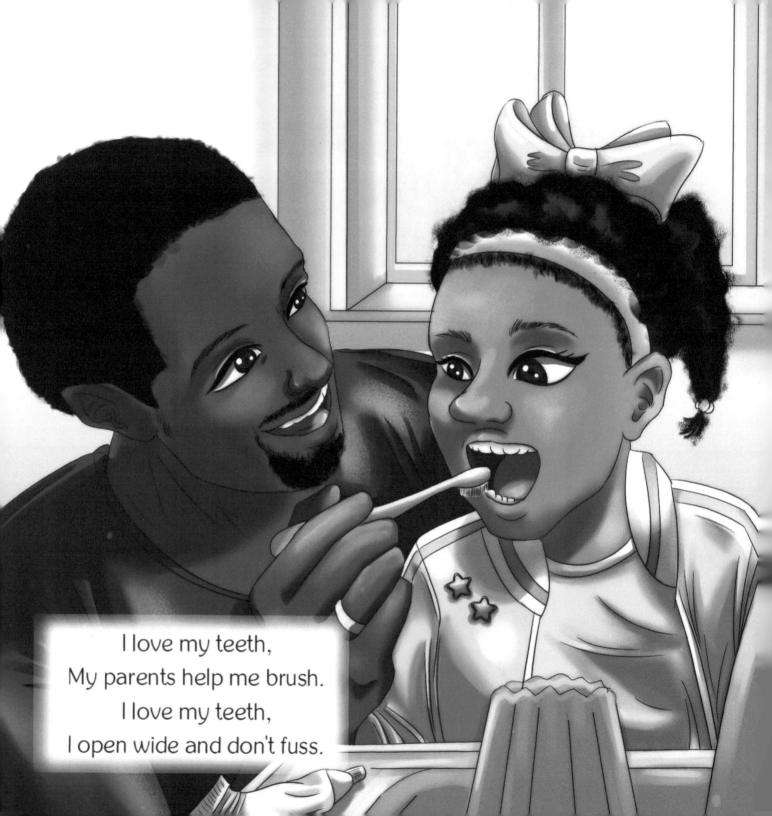

I love my teeth,
My parents help me brush.
I love my teeth,
I open wide and don't fuss.

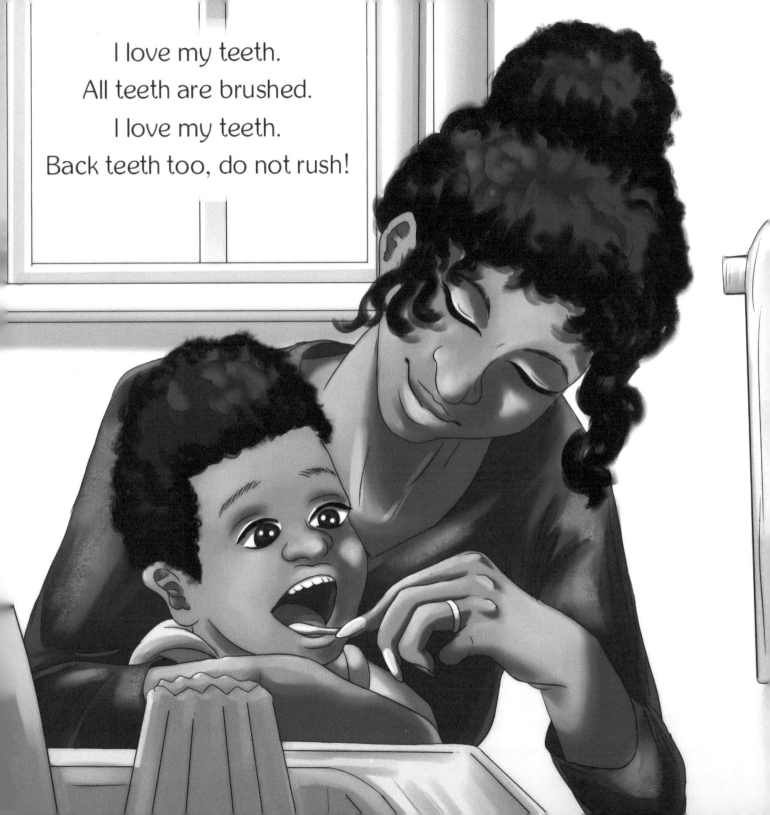

I love my teeth.
All teeth are brushed.
I love my teeth.
Back teeth too, do not rush!

I love my teeth.

But cannot forget my tongue.

I brush the top once or twice.

And then I am done.

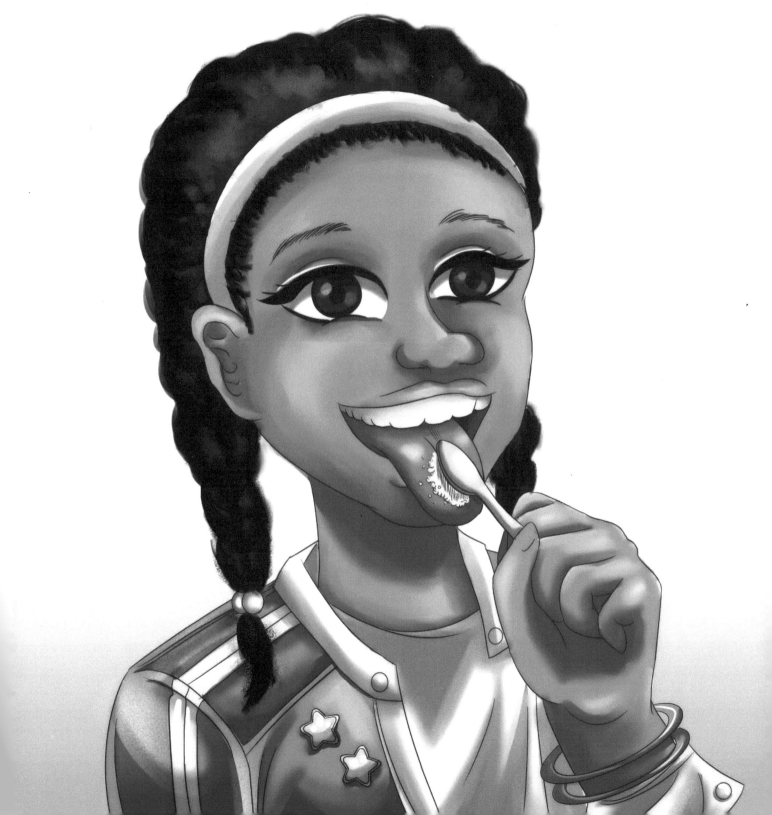

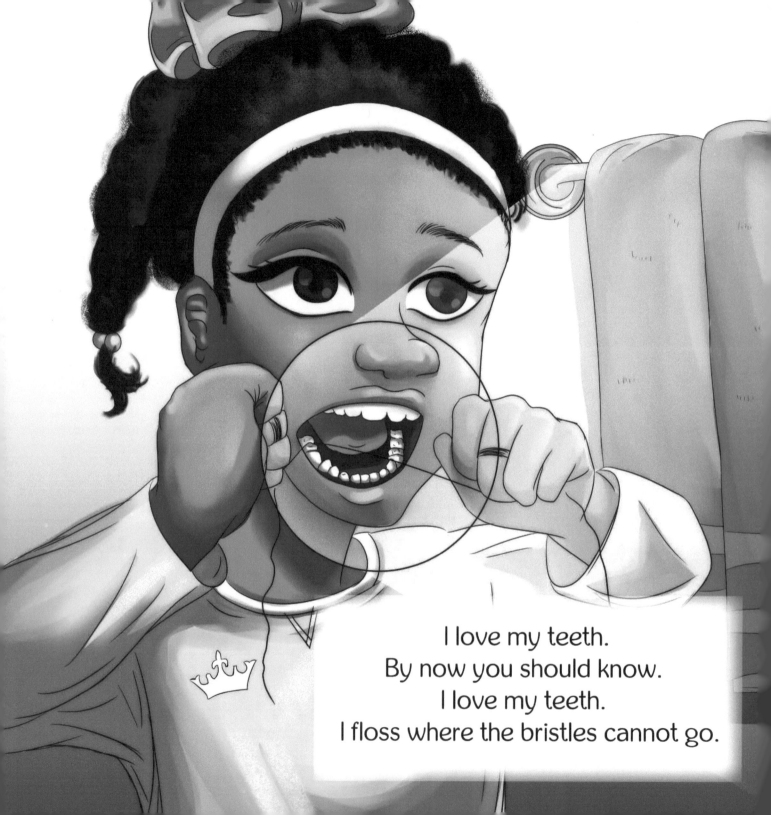

I love my teeth.
By now you should know.
I love my teeth.
I floss where the bristles cannot go.

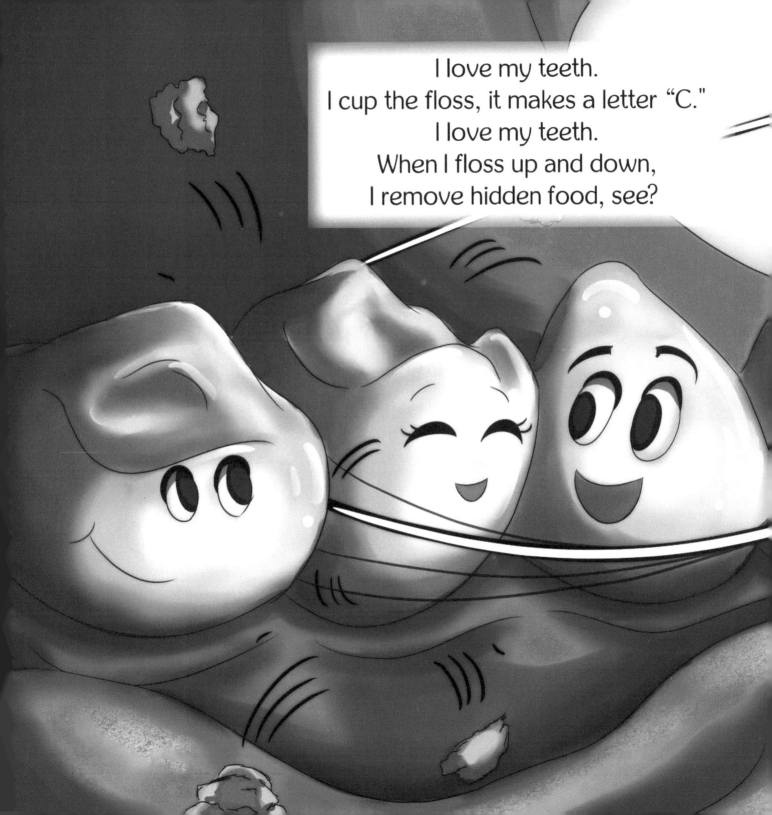

I love my teeth.
Now they are bright pearly white.
I love my teeth.
They help me eat what I like.

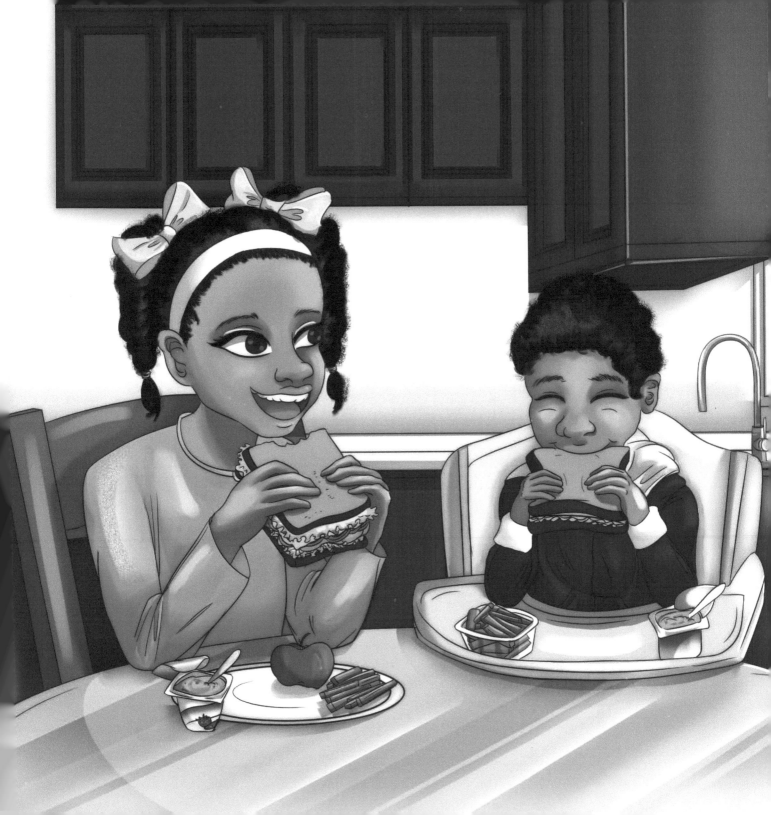

I love my teeth.
So, I eat healthy food.
I love my teeth.
Too many sweets…

Puts them in a bad mood.

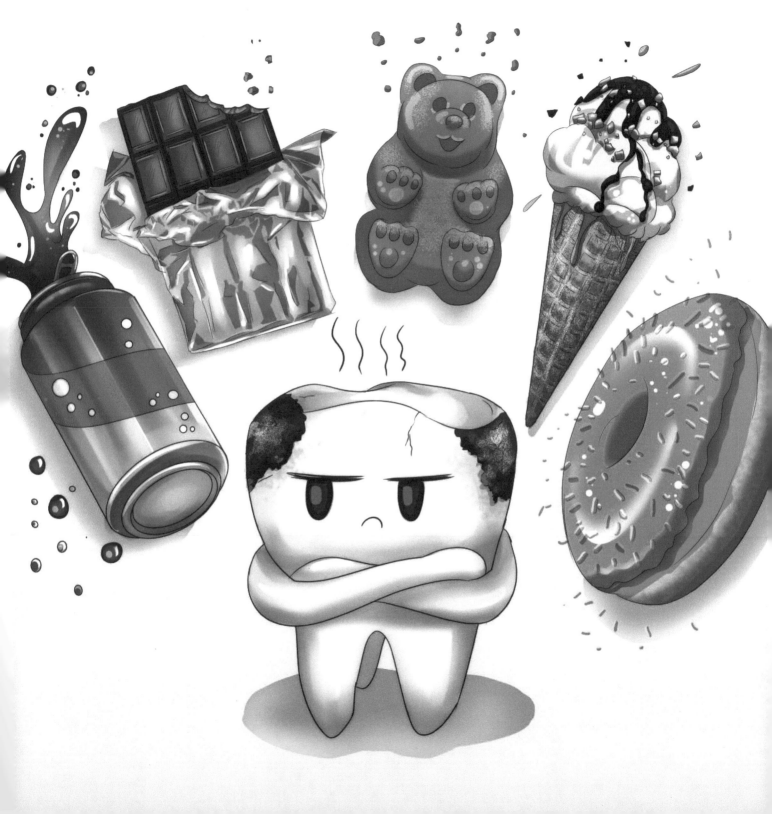

I love my teeth.
I drink lots of water.
I take care of my teeth.
My dental visits are shorter!

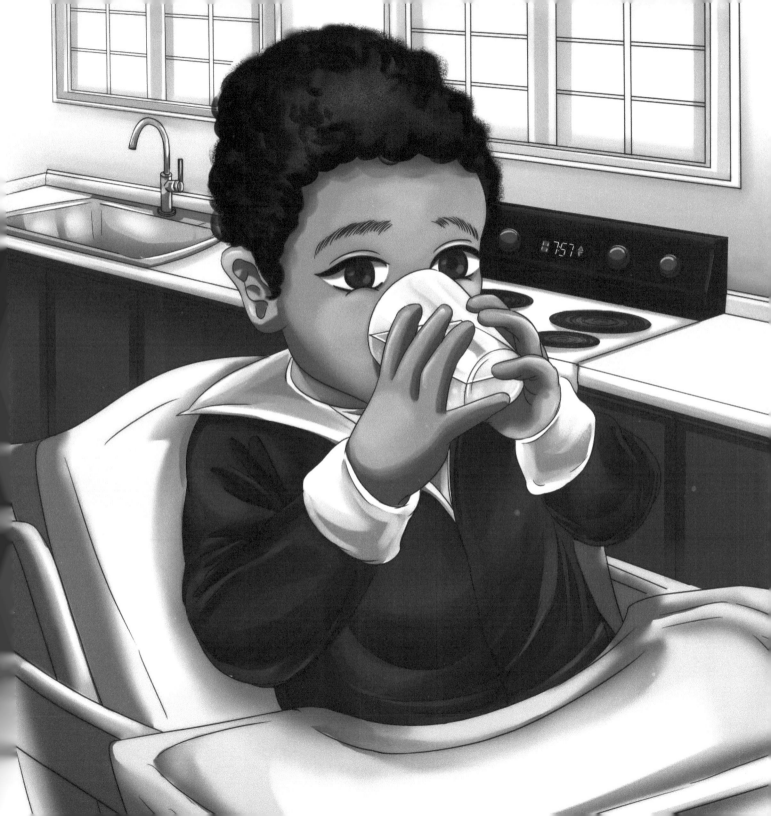

I love my teeth.
When playing sports
I wear a mouthpiece.

I love my teeth.
The dentist makes it fit
perfectly for me!

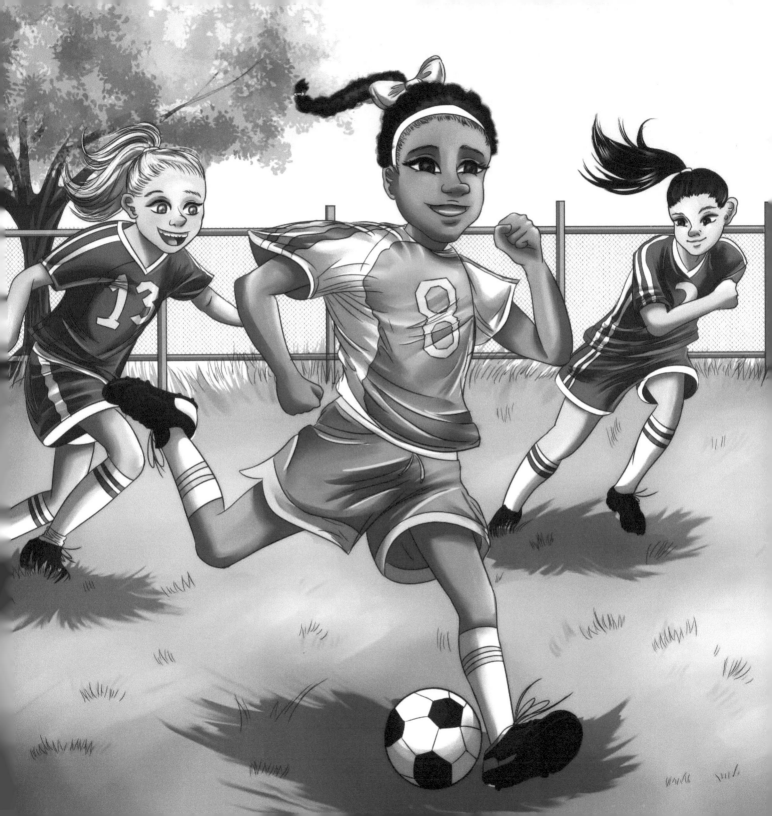

I love my teeth.

I care for them every day.

I love my teeth.

Cavity-free they will stay!

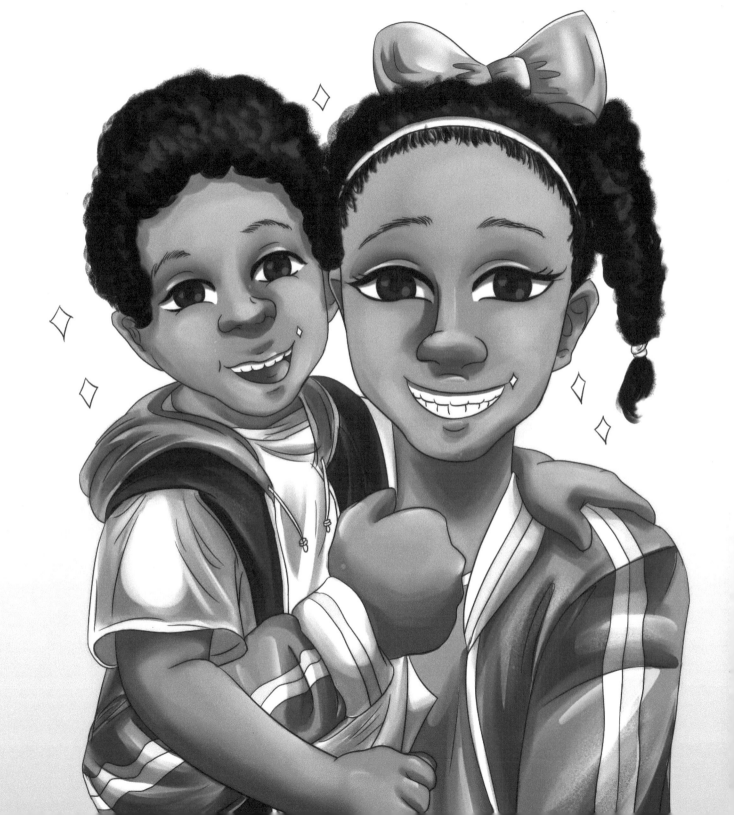

About the Author

Deveda Jackson became passionate about children's oral health after working several years as a Dental Hygienist in a pediatric dental office. However, her love for dentistry evolved growing up observing and working for her father who is a dentist. She graduated from James Madison University with a Bachelor's of Science degree in Biology, then obtained a second degree in Dental Hygiene from Old Dominion University. Deveda is a wife and mother of two bright, young children.

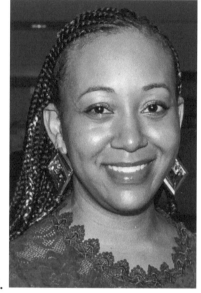

While working in a pediatric office, Deveda saw numerous children as young as 1 and 2 years old with a mouthful of cavities. This was disheartening to her because many of the kids reminded her of her own children. It was clear that a lot of her patients were not taught how to properly care for their teeth and gums. In addition, they did not understand how having poor oral health as a child can affect them for the rest of their life. She saw a need to teach children and their parents proper oral care by becoming an author focusing on children's oral health. Deveda hopes this book will educate kids and parents on how to take care of their teeth and build good habits early enough to prevent dental issues throughout their life.

CPSIA information can be obtained
at www.ICGtesting.com
Printed in the USA
BVHW010010090123
655867BV00002B/49

9 798986 383101